AF077510

DEPRESSION:
Don't Let It Get You Down

Help From: Basic Medical

Personal Experience

Scriptures From The Holy Bible

C. William Sorrels, PD

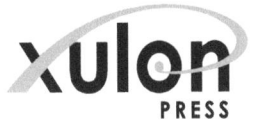

Copyright © 2016 by C. William Sorrels, PD

Depression: Don't Let It Get You Down
Help From: Basic Medical Personal Experience Scriptures From The Holy Bible
by C. William Sorrels, PD

Printed in the United States of America.

ISBN 9781498492249

All rights reserved solely by the author. The author guarantees all contents are original and do not infringe upon the legal rights of any other person or work. No part of this book may be reproduced in any form without the permission of the author. The views expressed in this book are not necessarily those of the publisher.

Unless otherwise indicated, Scripture quotations taken from the New King James Version (NKJV). Copyright © 1979, 1980, 1982 by Thomas Nelson, Inc. Used by permission. All rights reserved.

Scripture quotations taken from the New Living Translation (NLT). Copyright © 1996, 2004, 2007 by Tyndale House Foundation. Used by permission. All rights reserved.

www.xulonpress.com

Dedication

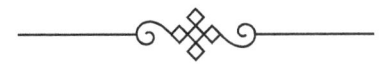

This book is dedicated to my dear, sweet wife, Mary Ann, who never wavered in her love, prayers or support for me or in her faith. She trusted that God would protect her and me from the satanic attacks and bring us closer to Him through it all. Amen!

Table Of Contents

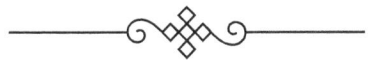

Introduction		ix
I.	Chapter One: The Dream	13
II.	Chapter Two: Causes of Depression	17
III.	Chapter Three: Treatment for Depression	27
IV.	Chapter Four: The Proof of the Truth of God's Word	41
V.	Chapter Five: Help from God's Word	49
VI.	Chapter Six: My Three Depressions and What God Taught Me	59
VII.	Chapter Seven: God Loves You	79
References		83

Introduction

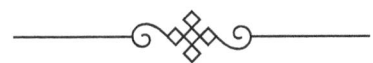

I have written this book in an attempt to help people who are struggling in and through the dungeon of depression. I do not claim to be an authority on this subject as this was not my field of study, but I do have the following credentials for writing such a book.
1. As a practicing pharmacist of thirty-nine years, and still in practice two days a week, I have dealt with and tried to help hundreds of depressed patients through the years. That included counseling with them and answering their questions about their medications and the importance of following their doctors' directions and seeing the results when they didn't.
2. I have suffered through three separate episodes of depression myself and therefore can speak to the subject from those personal experiences.
3. I am a Bible-believing Christian who has read and studied God's Word daily for many, many years. I have experienced the Bible's life-changing power in my life

and have seen it in the lives of others. I have also witnessed its ability to defeat the devil, in his attempts to destroy our lives.

Therefore, trusting Christ my Savior to guide me in the writing of this book, I have compiled information from several sources and combined that with my own personal experiences. This I have done in an attempt to bring to you, the reader, information to help you deal with your *Depression* and *Not Let It Get You Down*! To God be the Glory!

Of major importance: at the first signs or symptoms of depression, you *must* talk to your doctor, or mental health specialist, and schedule an appointment. (See the Mayo Clinic statement below.) Depression is not something to fool around with; it can be very serious and has detrimental consequences for the patient, and for other people around them. It can usually be treated and controlled, with very little or no disruption of normal life. Your doctor can determine if you need medication or not. It is important that you stay in close contact with your doctor and follow his/her instructions carefully. You must take your medication (if prescribed) correctly and not discontinue or change the dose without discussing that with your doctor, and then only according to his/her instructions. You must report to your doctor any changes in how you feel or what's going through your head.

Introduction

This statement is from the website of The Mayo Clinic:

When to see a doctor – If you feel depressed, make an appointment to see your doctor as soon as you can. If you're reluctant to seek treatment, talk to a friend or loved one, a health care professional, a faith leader, or someone else you trust.

When to get emergency help – If you think you may hurt yourself or attempt suicide, call 911 or your local emergency number immediately. Also consider these options if you're having suicidal thoughts:
- Call your mental health specialist.
- Call a suicide hotline number – in the U.S., call the National Suicide Prevention Lifeline at 1-800-273-TALK (1-800-273-8255). Use that same number and press "1" to reach the Veterans Crisis Line.
- Seek help from your primary doctor or other health care provider.
- Reach out to a close friend or loved one.
- Contact a minister, spiritual leader or someone else in your faith community.[5]

Of eternal importance: my greatest prayer for you is that if you don't know Jesus Christ as your Lord and Savior, and you're not a hundred percent sure where you will go when you die, that you will come to know Him and be known by Him. Chapter 7 can guide you, as it contains The Road Map to Heaven!

Chapter One
The Dream

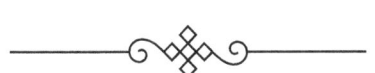

Shortly after my third depression God revealed to me the meaning of a recurring dream I experienced as a child. Travel back with me to the mid-1950s when I was five or six years old. At that time, I experienced a very disturbing dream. Actually it was a nightmare. I can't remember now how often it occurred, but I do remember it scared me every time. When I would wake I would bail out of my bed and hit the floor running to jump into my parents' bed. When I did this I was not always welcome, and sometimes they would march me back to my bed. But when it was "the dream," they always let me stay. They would comfort me and calm me down as I would usually be crying.

You may think some hideous monster was chasing me or snakes were invading my bed, or my plate of spaghetti had attacked me and was wrapping around my neck to choke me. It was nothing like that. In the dream I would be suspended in the air, above earth but not all the way in space. Nothing was above me but the twinkling stars against an early evening darkening sky, not totally black.

Somewhere way up above me was a man chopping wood. I couldn't see him very well, but he was big with a full beard and dressed like a lumberjack. From where I was, he looked pretty mean and ugly. He was chopping logs off a big tree trunk with a large, sharp ax. The tree had already been chopped down and all the limbs cleared from it, and the logs were about the size that would go into a large fireplace. Each log would come hurtling right at me, as if for some reason he was hoping they would conk me and do me in.

Being suspended in mid-air, it was extremely difficult to get out of the way. I would paddle with my hands and kick with my feet and legs as if I were in water, but that didn't work very well against air. I hardly seemed to move at all, but somehow each log missed me and would go speeding past me. The logs were different sizes, some large, some small, some in between, but all headed right at me, one at a time and not close together. As you can imagine, this was very frightening. Each one looked as though it would knock me out—or worse—and my efforts to move out of the way seemed futile. But they always missed. Some came very close to me as I could feel the wind when they whooshed by, while others were an elbow's length away, and still others an arm's length away.

I don't know how long the dream lasted, but it seemed a long time. I know now most dreams are very short in real

The Dream

time; the dream time seems long, but I think in real time they only last a few seconds. When I would wake up, my heart would be pounding, and I would seem worn out from all the paddling. I really wasn't, but it certainly seemed that way. That's when I would hit the floor and run to my parents' room, usually blubbering and crying.

After a while the dream became less often, but as far as I can remember it always scared me, and I never came to realize that none of the logs would hit me. Then without really noticing I realized one day that I wasn't having that dream anymore. I couldn't remember when I'd had the last one, but I was very thankful it was gone.

Some fifty-seven years later, God revealed to me the interpretation of the dream. I don't believe all dreams have a meaning; but I discovered this one did, and it brought peace to me when the Lord opened its meaning to me. Later in this book I will reveal the interpretation.

Chapter Two
Causes Of Depression

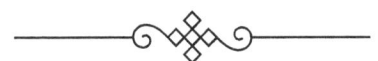

"Anxiety in the heart of man
causes depression."
Proverbs 12:25a

The brain is an organ just like every other organ in our bodies, and in the same manner as the other organs it can get sick. And because a sick brain can affect our thoughts, emotions and actions, the ramifications of a sick brain can be devastating to the individual and to people around us.[1] Also a stigma goes with a sick brain. If your heart is sick, you just have a bad heart; if your liver is sick, you have a bad liver; but if your brain is sick, you are crazy. That terminology is very demeaning to individuals who have a sick brain, and I am thankful it is being used less and less. Mental illness is an increasing problem in our society today, and there are many reasons for that. But this is not a medical book, so I will not attempt to cover everything.

As with all the organs in our bodies, the brain has specific functions. The cells that do the work in the brain are neurons. We are able to perceive the world, think and solve problems, form and retrieve memories, plan and carry out our intentions and actions, generate emotions and moods, due to complex interacting networks of these neurons as they send and receive messages. Our brain is more complex than any computer system we could ever design and weighs about three pounds with a hundred billion neurons.[1]

The brain chemicals of emotions and moods are called neurotransmitters, which facilitate the passage of signals from one neuron to another. There are several of these neuroamines, as they are also called, but the main three involved in stress, anxiety and depression are serotonin, norepinephrine and dopamine. These three neuroamines are involved in regulation of mood, emotions, sleep, arousal, attention, movement and feelings of pleasure. High levels of two basic emotions, fear and sadness, can result from abnormalities in the levels of these three chemicals.[1] As a practicing pharmacist, I dispense a number of different antidepressant medications every day, the majority of which have their pharmacological effect by increasing available brain levels of serotonin, norepinephrine and/or dopamine.

What exactly is depression? The Mayo Clinic gives the following definition:

Causes Of Depression

Depression is a mood disorder that causes a persistent feeling of sadness and loss of interest. Also called major depressive disorder or clinical depression, it affects how you feel, think and behave and can lead to a variety of emotional and physical problems. You may have trouble doing normal day-to-day activities, and sometimes you may feel as if life isn't worth living.

More than just a bout of the blues, depression isn't a weakness and you can't simply "snap out" of it. Depression may require long-term treatment. But don't get discouraged. Most people with depression feel better with medication, psychological counseling or both.[5]

Symptoms of depression can vary from person to person depending on many factors, but depression is not just being sad for a few days. The low mood will last from weeks to years with the potential to disrupt every aspect of the person's life. Some may not be able to leave the house or even get out of bed, while others may be restless, irritable or even agitated and angry. Some sleep too much while others have difficulty sleeping; some overeat while others are seldom hungry. Over time the symptoms may change, getting better or worse, or even disappear.[1]

Many subtypes of depression exist, of which one is dysthymia. This word comes from a Greek term meaning "bad state of mind." It describes a low grade of depression where the depressed mood doesn't reach the severity of depression. The person with dysthymia may feel depressed a lot of the day but can still carry out normal daily activities of living and work. Formal treatment, however, is usually necessary. Although not as severe as depression it can still be somewhat disabling.[1] And if this is you, you should report it to your doctor. Your doctor must be the one to decide if you need medication, or if you may do well on other practical means, and you can discuss this with your doctor. I have included some practical means in Chapter 3, and in the last part of Chapter 6 I discuss what I learned and what God taught me. The items listed there helped me greatly and may help you as well.

On the other hand, a very severe form of depression is psychotic depression in which the depression is so deep the person may lose contact with reality on occasions. This can bring on distorted thought processes, hallucinations and delusions. This can result in the hearing of voices (auditory hallucinations), thinking you've committed an imaginary crime or that your organs are rotting, or many other such imaginary things.[1] When these types of thoughts come, and/or thoughts of suicide or harming another person or people, this can create a vicious cycle of fear to anxiety to depression to distorted thoughts to fear to anxiety to depression and so on.

Depression has no one single cause. Many factors may combine to bring on a depressive disorder, including biological, psychological, social, chemical and structural changes in the brain, genetic vulnerability, cognitive and emotional functioning, and stressful life events. Other factors include early life stress and learned thinking patterns. Of all these factors, chronic stress may be the single most powerful cause of depression.[1]

Occasional stress or transient emotional states are not usually a strong predictor of depression. A personal example will take us back to when I was around nine years old and into mischief with my two brothers. Our mom came into the room unnoticed, and suddenly a hand from nowhere had my older brother and me by the hair of our heads. Our younger brother, who was the instigator of the whole thing, scurried behind a chair. Obviously all action stopped. When your mom has you by your hair, you have no recourse but to be still. Each of us was ordered to our room, and then we heard those words we never wanted to hear: "Wait there until your father gets home!"

Analysis of situation when you reached your room:

First stress: Hair grasped by someone you didn't even know was in the room, an immediate indication that you're caught fighting with your brothers, which you are forbidden to do. Daddy always said enough was against us out in the world so we should never be against each other.

Second stress: Ordered to room creating an uncertain outcome. At this point, however, the stress level is not too bad since being sent to your room usually didn't bring about any pain—just hurt your feelings some.

Third and major stress: Those words "Wait until your father gets home" always brought a significant level of stress, exhibited by anxiety, fear, trepidation and woeful expectation. Now the pain could be real from a pounding on our posterior that would be more than just uncomfortable. (Our father never spanked us anywhere but on our bottom and never left marks. He was quite talented in knowing just how much pressure to apply to get our attention!) But pain, agony and tears usually resulted.

I considered my options.

1. Run! Get outta there. Go out the window and climb the nearest tall tree and stay there until Daddy goes to work the next morning. Probable outcome: much worse situation, stinging posterior pain, probable loss of outdoor playing privileges for a long while and no ice cream forever!
2. Blame my brothers and explain that I was only a victim of their misbehavior. Probable outcome: worse situation since Daddy is not fooled. I would be caught lying and experience a similar but not as severe outcome as option 1.
3. Cry profusely, confess and ask Daddy for mercy; repent and promise never to do it again. Possible outcome:

forgiveness granted with possibly no posterior pain and lighter punishment, although we would receive punishment of some kind. Stress level starts to subside but doesn't disappear completely until mercy applied.

So these transient, emotional states are something we all deal with. We can all feel down, or what we call 'depressed', over this situation or that, but clinical depression is different. The Merriam-Webster Dictionary gives the following full definition for depression:
1. A state of feeling sad: dejection
2. A psychoneurotic or psychotic disorder marked especially by sadness, inactivity, difficulty in thinking and concentration, a significant increase or decrease in appetite and time spent sleeping, feelings of dejection and hopelessness, and sometimes suicidal tendencies.[7]

Chronic stress, however, can produce thoughts of helplessness and hopelessness as one deals with day-in and day-out multiple stressors, especially over a long period of time. These types of thoughts can promote and sustain a mood of depression. Also, people who are experiencing chronic stress tend not to take care of themselves very well. They don't eat properly or exercise and may smoke or drink to excess. This type of lifestyle can further increase the likelihood of developing depression.[1]

The following is a list of other things that can cause or trigger depression.[1] I won't list every single thing or give a complete explanation of each one.

1. Childhood abuse can greatly disrupt the stress system and escalate the risk for depression.

2. Heritage may be a factor as several genes have been identified that affect the risk for depression.

3. Poor diet has definitely been linked to increasing the likelihood for depression. More than one study has associated a diet high in fast foods and other foods high in trans-fatty acids with depression.

4. Other lifestyle factors such as overwork, lack of physical exercise and even where you live have been linked to developing or aggravating depression symptoms.

5. Hundreds of studies have connected chronic pain to developing depression, as pain can affect thoughts, moods, memory, attention and behavior. This may lead to depression risk factors such as isolation, immobility and possible drug addiction.

6. Medical illnesses and medications may be responsible for up to twenty percent of all depressions. Chronic illness is a definite high risk factor for developing depression, and many medications can cause or contribute to depression symptoms.

I have been diagnosed with obsessive-compulsive disorder (OCD) which can contribute to developing depression. The Mayo Clinic staff defines OCD as being "characterized by unreasonable thoughts and fears (obsessions) that lead you to do repetitive behaviors (compulsions). It's also possible to have only obsessions or only compulsions and still have OCD." Additional problems or complications linked to OCD include anxiety disorders, depression and overall poor quality of life.[5] Therefore, it is quite easy to see how this disease can contribute to developing or aggravating symptoms of depression.

7. Age can be a major factor although depression can develop during childhood, adolescence and old age. The symptoms of a major depressive disorder are usually first seen in adulthood and highest in the thirties and forties. The prevalence in eighteen- to twenty-nine-year-olds is three-fold higher than folks over sixty.

8. A prevailing mood state called subjective well-being or life satisfaction. Avoiding a continual pessimistic mood state can be highly important in NOT developing depression.

9. Substance abuse can also lead to episodes of depression.

We live in an uncertain world—a complex, cultural environment—and each of us will encounter different stressors of one kind or another on a regular basis. Nothing is certain anymore, other than the promises of God. We hear of wars and rumors of wars; natural disasters are on the rise; strange viruses are popping up, causing weird diseases; the family is attacked on all sides, creating instability in the home and in the raising of children; financial collapses occur; and the list goes on. Obviously, all this increases fear, anxiety and depression.

Evil is on the rise. If you read the newspaper or watch the news, there is no news like bad news. And not only that, evil is promoted throughout our culture. Movies, television, advertisements, video games, magazines and the like all promote evil, and people buy it. Evil creates fear, anxiety and depression.

We do it to ourselves, by doing things we know are wrong. For example, you're cheating on your husband or wife, and you're concerned you'll get caught. Or you're embezzling from your employer, and you're afraid he'll find out. All of these things can cause fear, anxiety and depression.

Worry. Worry is a definite cause for depression, as it creates fear and anxiety, which of course can result in depression. Statistics have shown the following facts about worry: forty percent of the things we worry about never happen; thirty percent of those worries are about things in the past, which now we can't do anything about; twelve percent of our worries are concerns about our health, even when we're not sick; ten percent of the worries we have are about friends/neighbors and usually based on conjecture. That leaves only eight percent of our worries with any possibility of actually happening![2]

Chapter Three
Treatment For Depression

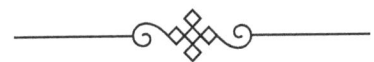

** You read the following paragraph, and the statement from The Mayo Clinic in the introduction, but I have also included them here because of their importance, and in case you are dealing with thoughts of suicide, or harming yourself or someone else. **

Of major importance: at the first signs or symptoms of depression, you must talk to your doctor or mental health specialist and schedule an appointment. (See the Mayo Clinic statement below.) Depression is not something to fool around with; it can be very serious and have detrimental consequences for the patient, and for other people around them. It can usually be treated and controlled with very little or no disruption of normal life. Your doctor can determine if you need medication or not. It is important that you stay in close contact with your doctor, and follow his/her instructions carefully. You must take your medication (if prescribed) correctly and *not* discontinue or change the dose without discussing that with your doctor, and then only according to his/her instructions. You must report to your doctor any changes in how you feel or what's going through your head.

This statement is from the website of The Mayo Clinic:

When to see a doctor–If you feel depressed, make an appointment to see your doctor as soon as you can. If you're reluctant to seek treatment, talk to a friend or loved one, a health care professional, a faith leader, or someone else you trust.

When to get emergency help–If you think you may hurt yourself or attempt suicide, call 911 or your local emergency number immediately! Also consider these options if you're having suicidal thoughts:

- Call your mental health specialist
- Call a suicide hotline number – in the U.S., call the National Suicide Prevention Lifeline at 1-800-273-TALK (1-800-273-8255). Use that same number and press "1" to reach the Veterans Crisis Line.
- Seek help from your primary doctor or other health care provider.
- Reach out to a close friend or loved one.
- Contact a minister, spiritual leader or someone else in your faith community.[5]

Remember, your doctor, preferably a mental health specialist, must determine whether you need medications or other treatments, or not. However, as the following items are listed as contributing to a depressed state, obviously making changes to eliminate or lessen these should help to lessen or eliminate symptoms:

1. Poor diet and not drinking enough water (eat a balanced diet, including enough water).
2. Overworked (slow down; don't be a workaholic).
3. Lack of physical exercise (start walking; get an exercise bike or treadmill; join a gym). NOTE- if you haven't been exercising, you must start out slow.
4. A prevailing, pessimistic mood state (try to develop and keep a positive attitude; talk to friends who will encourage you).
5. Evil (don't watch the violent, sensual, blood and guts movies and TV shows, or read books that are filled with the same, or play violent video games).
6. Worry (worry accomplishes nothing; send worries and fears up to the Lord. See Chapter 5 and 6 on more about handling worry, and Chapter 7 to find out how to be right with God in God's eyes).
7. Stress (make changes where possible to eliminate or lessen your level of stress).

In the United States today the most common way a major depressive disorder is treated is by medications called

antidepressants. Several different classes of antidepressant medications are separated by how they work in the body. Following is a list of some of the classes[1]:
 * SSRI–Selective Serotonin Re-uptake Inhibitors
 * SNRI–Serotonin-Norepinephrine Re-uptake Inhibitors
 * NDRI–Norepinephrine-Dopamine Re-uptake inhibitors
 * TCAs–Tricyclic Antidepressants
 * MAOI–Monoamine Oxidase Inhibitors
 * Re-uptake Inhibitors and Receptor Blockers

Also anti-anxiety and antipsychotic medications may be prescribed for depressed patients.

Of all these meds the most commonly prescribed for depression are the SSRIs, or Selective Serotonin Re-uptake Inhibitors. Generally, they are thought to have fewer side effects than the other classes as a whole, but as in all the classes the response can vary greatly from patient to patient. Therefore, no one class seems to stand out above the others in effectiveness. And, unfortunately, the best way to find out which medication or combination of medications is right for a certain patient is usually trial and error.[1]

It should be noted that all medications, from aspirin to chemotherapy, can have side effects, but the percentages of patients who experience side effects is usually very low. Your doctor can determine if the benefit outweighs the risk, and you can discuss that with him/her. Also of note on these types of medications is that they don't work immediately.

Treatment For Depression

As I mentioned before, most of these medications work by increasing available levels of three main neurotransmitters—serotonin, norepinephrine and/or dopamine—in the brain. The medication may actually change the level of these brain chemicals within an hour or less, but it is normally several weeks before the patient gets relief from the symptoms.

Animal and human studies have revealed why this is generally the case. In order for the medication to help alleviate symptoms, three things normally must take place within the brain: 1. Processes within the neuron must be stimulated; 2. The number of neurons in the hippocampus and other places must be increased; 3. More connections between neurons must be created. These types of neuronal changes may take several weeks to happen. This doesn't mean that some relief won't occur earlier than that, as it will. But a maximum effect usually takes several weeks.[1]

Please note from the previous three paragraphs important points about these medications: 1. It may take trial and error by your prescriber to get the right medication or combination of medications for you. 2. It may take a few weeks to get maximum relief from your symptoms.

Many other treatments are available for depression, but your mental health provider will inform you about those if he or she deems it necessary.

Other things can help maintain good health, both physical and mental, including[1]:

* Learn to relax

* Change negative thinking to positive
* Maintain a good healthy diet; low levels of vitamin B12, folate and vitamin D have been linked to increased levels of depression, as the B vitamins have been shown to help regulate mood while vitamin D helps neuronal communications.
* Fish and krill oils have been shown to be crucial for good brain function but have inconsistent results in helping depression.
* Exercise and physical activity have been shown, by many studies, to have beneficial effects on depression symptoms. A half hour to an hour of moderate exercise like brisk walking is recommended on all or most days of the week.

I recommend you read your Bible daily, and spend time in prayer. This is discussed in more detail in later chapters.

Here credit should be given where credit is due. All healing comes from God. God is sovereign, and nothing would work if He didn't ordain it. No medicine, no surgery, no procedure, no treatments of any kind would work except He allow it. And that's not a new thing; it's always been that way.

Even when Jesus walked the earth, He may not have healed everyone with whom He came in contact. In the Bible in the Gospel of John, chapter 5, verses 2-3a and 5-9, we read about Jesus coming into an area by the Sheep Gate in

Jerusalem where there was a multitude of sick people. He looked down at one guy, who had been crippled for thirty-eight years, and told him to get up, pick up his bed and walk, which the man did. There is no record of Jesus healing anyone else in that area that day, although He could have. Other scriptures tell us Jesus did heal everyone brought to Him at that particular time, as in Matthew 4:24: "Then His fame went throughout all Syria; and they brought to Him all sick people who were afflicted with various diseases and torments, and those who were demon-possessed, epileptics, and paralytics; and He healed them."

An example of someone actually calling out to the Lord for healing but not being healed is the apostle Paul in 2 Corinthians 12:7-10: "...Even though I have received such wonderful revelations from God. So to keep me from becoming proud, I was given a thorn in my flesh, a messenger from Satan to torment me and keep me from becoming proud. Three different times I begged the Lord to take it away. Each time he said, 'My grace is all you need. My power works best in weakness.' So now I am glad to boast about my weaknesses, so that the power of Christ can work through me. That's why I take pleasure in my weaknesses, and in the insults, hardships, persecutions, and troubles that I suffer for Christ. For when I am weak, then I am strong" (NLT). And this same apostle Paul, whose thorn in the flesh God did not remove, was given divine revelation and visions and wrote a number of books in the New Testament. His response to not being healed is the correct response for all of us who have to deal with physical challenges. Never easy, but always the correct response.

Although we can't always understand why some people are healed while others are not, we know God is in control and allows healing or not depending on His will. His divine purposes may be better served by allowing sickness or injury in some instances. Sometimes God may allow what He hates in order to accomplish what He loves. But, by all means, we pray for those who are sick and trust God for the outcome.

Therefore, God heals directly (supernatural) and indirectly (medical treatment or some other means), and it's always been that way and still is today. Because of all the amazing technology God has allowed in these days, we see the indirect healing more than the direct. But God still heals both ways, and it's always He who does the healing.

The following are some examples of indirect healing in God's Word:

* "Is anyone among you sick? Let him call for the elders of the church, and let them pray over him, anointing him with oil in the name of the Lord. And the prayer of faith will save the sick, and the Lord will raise him up" (James 5:14-15a). It should be noted that it is the Lord's intervention that does the healing, not the oil or the elders or their faith.[2] In biblical times oil was considered to have medicinal value or was sacramental, but many see it as a symbol of the Holy Spirit's healing power falling upon the sick person. "In the name of the Lord" strictly indicates it is God, not the oil, that heals.[6]

* "When He had said these things, He spat on the ground and made clay with the saliva; and anointed the eyes of the blind man with the clay. And He said to him, 'Go, wash in the pool of Siloam' (which is translated, Sent). So he went and washed, and came back seeing" (John 9:6-7). Jesus, of course, is the one who is speaking to the blind man, and He could have just spoken the word and the man would be able to see. But here, for some reason, probably to test the man's faith and build his trust in Christ, Christ uses an apparent indirect method.

* "So he went to him and bandaged his wounds, pouring on oil and wine; and he set him on his own animal, brought him to an inn, and took care of him" (Luke 10:34). This is found in the story of the good Samaritan (see Luke 10:30-37). A man was beaten and robbed and left for dead, and although a priest and a Levite wouldn't stop to help him, a man from Samaria did. It indicates typical medical treatment for that day for someone who had been beaten. The story seems to indicate that the man recovers by indirect means, even though he was left half dead.

As far as supernatural or miraculous healing goes, I will share what happened to me in the fall of 1989. In the previous

November, God had called me to serve Him in The Gideons International. My wife, Mary Ann, also felt the call and joined the Auxiliary of The Gideons International. The Gideons International has one purpose, and that is to see that every person on earth has an opportunity to receive Jesus Christ as Lord and Savior. We do that mainly by personal evangelism and placing the Word of God, the Holy Bible.

At that time, I was working as a pharmacist at a small retail pharmacy. Occasionally I would cover a hospital pharmacy (where I used to work) on a weekend for their regular pharmacist, usually just on Sunday. I would work extra on Sunday for two reasons: one, to make extra money, and, two, so I wouldn't be available to serve the Lord as He had called me to serve Him through the Gideon ministry.

Early that fall I had worked in the hospital pharmacy three Sundays in a row and came down with mononucleosis. This also resulted in having hepatitis. I was one sick dude. I had what seemed like fuzzy stuff down in my throat that I couldn't spit out or swallow. It was just there. It felt like hairy peanut butter. It was awful. I felt bad for three weeks and missed at least a whole week of work and had to take a number of medications.

A few weeks after that I worked another three Sundays and came down with cat scratch fever. One of our cats had scratched me on the palm of my left hand, and shortly the lymph nodes under my left arm became swollen and painful. They just whomped up there, so I went to my doctor, was

Treatment For Depression

diagnosed with CSF, a bacterial infection, and was put on antibiotics. I didn't feel well for a couple of weeks but was thankful I did not have to miss any work.

Then, after working three or four Sundays around Thanksgiving, I developed a pain in my side. It was subtle at first, but it steadily worsened until it was very painful, even to barely touching it. I decided I should let a doctor check it out, so late one afternoon when we weren't busy at the pharmacy I walked across the street to the office of a surgeon who was a good friend and let him look me over. He examined me thoroughly. Shaking his head, he told me he was very sorry, but I had gall stones and they would need to come out.

This was bad news. I had already missed work earlier in the fall and didn't need to miss any more. Plus, I was between health insurances after changing jobs from the hospital to the retail pharmacy. This was early December, and my new health insurance wouldn't kick in until January 1. I did not have the time or the money to have surgery, but I knew I couldn't go on with this pain gnawing at my side. Perplexed, I walked back across the street to finish my day at the pharmacy.

It was about a forty-five-minute drive from the pharmacy to my home, most of which was on Interstate 40, and as I drove I prayed and discussed this situation with the Lord. I reminded the Lord—not that He needed reminding—of all the reasons I did not need to have surgery at this time. But I said, "Lord, I also can't go on with this terrible pain in my side either. O Lord, I need Your help!"

After crying out to the Lord and continuing to ponder the situation, without noticing it I was giving God time to speak to me. I did not hear an audible voice, but suddenly the whole picture came into clear focus. I could see what I had been doing, working on Sunday and making myself unavailable to speak in churches for the Gideon ministry. I was putting making money ahead of serving God who had called me with a loud voice to serve Him in the Gideons International. I hadn't had opportunities to speak on all those Sundays, but several of them I had. It was clear now God wanted me to be available on His schedule, not mine.

I confessed and repented before Him, and then I made a deal with the Lord. I'm not sure you should make a deal with the Lord, but it felt right at the time. And He has blessed it ever since. As I drove I prayed and said, "O Lord, please forgive me for not understanding or realizing what I have been doing. And humbly I thank You for your forgiveness and pledge this promise. If you will take this pain out of my side, I will never work another Sunday when it keeps me from speaking for You or serving You according to the call You have on my life."

After finishing the prayer I turned on the radio, and my thoughts drifted to other things. I had been home for about thirty minutes before I realized I was not hurting. I felt no pain in my side. I gently touched my side, no pain; I poked harder on my side, no pain; I pounded on my side with my fist, no pain. All the pain was gone!

I was overwhelmed. I dropped to my knees and thanked and praised the Lord Jesus and declared, "It's a deal!" And I continued praising Him and thanking Him for the miracle He had just wrought in me. That was in December 1989. The Lord has allowed me to remain faithful to that promise, and He has certainly kept His end of the bargain. I truly believe if I ever work on a Sunday and turn down an opportunity to speak for the Lord, I'll wind up with gall stones as big as golf balls. I'll finally hold a world record in something.

Chapter Four
The Proof Of The Truth Of God's Word

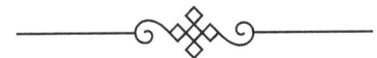

You may be wondering why I have included this chapter in a book on depression. It is simply because throughout the rest of this book, you will be reading many, many scriptures from the Bible, God's holy Word; and I want you to have an understanding of why we can believe in the Bible as the Word of God. It takes faith to believe in God, and it takes faith to believe in His Word. If you lack faith, God tells us, in His Word, how to develop faith; Romans 10:17: "So then faith comes by hearing, and hearing by the Word of God." However, I want you to understand that our faith is not a total leap into the dark, as you will see from the following information. We can find much help in God's Word to handle physical infirmities, and all trials and tribulations that come our way.

Throughout the centuries of time, critics have beat upon the Bible declaring it is not true and that it is only a book of fables and wonderful stories. Or parts of it are true, but it contains errors, contradictions and embellishment. Nothing could be further from the truth. This, I believe, is the bottom line. The Word of God reveals itself to be the true Word of God just as much as Jesus revealed Himself to be the Son of God. He walked on water, healed the lame, the lepers, the blind and the sick, raised the dead and resurrected from the dead. Most people didn't believe Him then, and most scoff at the Bible today. Why is this? Simple. They didn't like His message then, and they don't like many things the Bible says today. So, if you don't like the message, you just state that it's not true. That doesn't make it not true.

It should be noted that, due to the number of ancient manuscripts which have been found, we know with almost total accuracy what the original texts said. Also, where there is some question on the meaning of the original text, this never happens in Scripture verses that deal with vital elements of faith.[2]

The Bible is inspired, inerrant and authoritative. It cannot be authoritative if it is not inerrant (without errors), and there is no way it could be inerrant if man had written it.[2] Man likes to think he is that smart, but he is not.

Second Timothy 3:16 says, "All Scripture is given by inspiration of God and is profitable." The word "inspiration" comes from the Greek word *theopneustros*, which comes from *theos* (God) and *pneo* (to blow or breathe). Thus, the word "inspiration" means "breathed by God."[2]

Therefore, this means that the Spirit of God moved on the writers of the Scriptures as they wrote, so that each word penned came from Him and not from man. But this fact does not remove the distinctiveness, or style, of each author.[2]

Here are some amazing facts about the Bible.[3]

* Written over a fifteen-hundred-year span, which would be over forty generations.
* Written by some forty authors from all walks of life: Moses, a political leader trained in the universities of Egypt; Peter, a fisherman; Amos, a herdsman; Joshua, a military general; Nehemiah, a cup bearer; Daniel, a prime minister; Luke, a doctor; Solomon, a king; David, also a military general and a king; Matthew, a tax collector; Paul, a rabbi.
* Written in a number of diverse places, such as Moses in the wilderness, Jeremiah in a dungeon, Daniel on a hillside and in a palace, Paul inside prison walls, Luke while traveling, John on the Isle of Patmos; and David even wrote during his military campaigns.
* Some wrote from the heights of joy, while others wrote during deep sorrow and despair.
* Written on three continents, Asia, Africa and Europe, and in three languages, Hebrew, Aramaic and Greek.
* All Bible prophecy comes true exactly when it is supposed to. God records history in advance, and His accuracy rating is one hundred percent. For example, 322 Old Testament prophecies were fulfilled when

Christ was born (His first coming). The odds of that happening by pure chance are one in eighty-four followed by ninety-seven zeros! One of those prophecies is found in the book of Daniel, chapter 9. There Daniel predicts the triumphal entry of Christ into Jerusalem on a colt—and not just that, but also the very day it would occur. This was 483 years before it happened, and it happened on that very day 483 years later. At least two things are proven by all biblical prophecy coming true and exactly when predicted to do so: 1. God is the author of the Bible, and 2. God is the sovereign ruler of history.

Through all of this, amazingly, the overall theme is the same throughout: redemption, including creation, the fall, redemption and restoration. Many sub-themes are present, such as sin, forgiveness, salvation, love, eternity and the trinity, but the overall theme never changes.[2] It should be quite evident man could never put all of this together over fifteen hundred years by his own initiative, merit, creativity or wisdom.

And there are no errors or contradictions. Also, it should be noted that not one shovel of archaeologic dirt has ever contradicted the Bible. And, as time goes on, archaeology continues to verify scriptural information.

Throughout the years all attempts to destroy the Word of God have failed. The Roman emperor Nero, who beheaded the apostle Paul, attempted to rid the world of Christians and the Word of God, and he failed. Another Roman emperor, Diocletian, issued an edict in A.D. 303 to stop Christians from worshipping and to destroy their Scriptures. His edict failed, and only twenty-five years later the next Roman emperor, Constantine, declared that "fifty copies of the Scriptures would be prepared at the expense of the government."[3]

Also, it is a well-known fact that the infamous French writer, philosopher and atheist of the 1700s, Voltaire, made the following statement: "In one hundred years the Bible will be an extinct book." It is also well known that only fifty years after his death the Geneva Bible Society was using his house and his printing press to publish Bibles, and later his house was the Paris headquarters for the British and Foreign Bible Society. The indestructibility of the Bible greatly supports its infallibility.[4]

The fact is that no matter, no way, no how, will anyone ever destroy the Bible. Jesus makes that clear in Matthew 24:35 when He says, "Heaven and earth will pass away, but my words will never pass away."

Bernard Ramm, a Bible interpretation scholar, made this statement: "A thousand times over, the death knell of the Bible has been sounded, the funeral procession formed, the inscription cut on the tombstone and the committal read. But somehow the corpse never stays put. No other book has been so chopped, knifed, sifted, scrutinized and vilified...nor been subject to such venom and skepticism as the Bible. Yet today it is loved by millions, read by millions and studied by millions."³ It is still every year the number-one best-selling book in the world, and no other book is ever anywhere close.

In Psalm 19:7-11 we see what the Word of God can do for us.

> The law of the Lord is perfect, converting the soul; the testimony of the Lord is sure, making wise the simple; the statutes of the Lord are right, rejoicing the heart; the commandment of the Lord is pure, enlightening the eyes; the fear of the Lord is clean, enduring forever; the judgments of the Lord are true and righteous altogether. More to be desired are they than gold.... Moreover by them Your servant is warned, and in keeping them there is great reward.

To be considered also is the fact that the Word of God has the power to change the human heart. Jesus declares in the seventeenth chapter of John that only truth can sanctify (make holy) and that God's Word is the source of that truth.² As Jesus prays to His Father in John 17:17 He says, "Sanctify them by Your truth; Your Word is truth." He doesn't say it's almost true, true here but not there, or that each person reading it can determine for himself what's true and what isn't.

Dr. David Jeremiah, I believe, sums it up very well in a paragraph from his *Jeremiah Study Bible*. At the top of page 1722, under "For Reflection, Why We Need the Word," the final paragraph says, "Just as Jesus was fully man and fully God, the Bible is both a divine and human book. With Almighty God as its originator, it is completely true, without error in its original form, and thoroughly trustworthy."[2]

God's Word is true because God is true. And He is not some tiny, small god who could not control the writing of His book. The Bible is the inspired, inerrant, authoritative Word of God. Amen.

Chapter Five
Help From God's Word

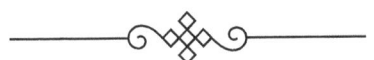

Please note that if you haven't already you should read chapter 4 before you read this chapter. These scriptures are taken out of the Bible, and chapter 4 helps you understand why we can trust the Word of God and what it tells us.

** See Chapter 7 to find out how to be right with God in God's eyes. **

I. HELP FROM THE OLD TESTAMENT

"The Lord is my shepherd; I shall not want. He makes me to lie down in green pastures; He leads me beside the still waters, He restores my soul; He leads me in the paths of righteousness for His name's sake. Yea, though I walk through the valley of the shadow of death, I will fear no evil; For You are with me; Your rod and Your staff, they comfort me. You prepare a table before me in the presence of my enemies; You anoint my head with oil; my cup runs over. Surely goodness and mercy shall follow me all the days of my life; and I will dwell in the house of the Lord forever." —Psalm 23

"For I know the thoughts that I think toward you, says the Lord, thoughts of peace and not of evil, to give you a future and a hope." —Jeremiah 29:11

"The Lord is my light and my salvation; whom shall I fear? The Lord is the strength of my life; of whom shall I be afraid?" —Psalm 27:1

"I sought the Lord, and He heard me, and delivered me from all my fears." —Psalm 34:4

"This poor man cried out, and the Lord heard him, and saved him out of all his troubles. The Angel of the Lord encamps all around those who fear (awesome respect) Him, and delivers them." —Psalm 34:6-7

"The eyes of the Lord are on the righteous, and his ears are open to their cry." —Psalm 34:15

"The righteous cry out, and the Lord hears, and delivers them out of all their troubles." —Psalm 34:17

"Many are the afflictions of the righteous, but the Lord delivers him out of them all." —Psalm 34:19

"God is our refuge and strength, a very present help in trouble. Therefore we will not fear, even though the earth be removed, and though the mountains be carried into the midst of the sea; though its waters roar and be troubled, though the mountains shake with its swelling." —Psalm 46:1-3

Help From God's Word

"Cast your burden on the Lord, and He shall sustain you."
—Psalm 55:22a

"Whenever I am afraid, I will trust in You." —Psalm 56:3

II. HELP FROM THE NEW TESTAMENT

Jesus is speaking, "Come to me, all you who labor and are heavy laden, and I will give you rest. Take My yoke upon you, and learn from Me, for I am gentle and lowly in heart, and you will find rest for your souls. For My yoke is easy and My burden is light." —Matthew 11:28-30

"For God has not given us a spirit of fear, but of power and of love and of a sound mind." —2 Timothy 1:7

"What then shall we say to these things? If God is for us, who can be against us?" —Romans 8:31

"Let your conduct be without covetousness; be content with such things as you have. For He Himself (God) has said, 'I will never leave you nor forsake you.' So we may boldly say: 'The Lord is my helper; I will not fear. What can man do to me?'" —Hebrews 13:5-6

"Therefore humble yourselves under the mighty hand of God, that He may exalt you in due time, casting all your care upon Him, for He cares for you." —1 Peter 5:6-7

"Be anxious for nothing, but in everything by prayer and supplication with thanksgiving, let your requests be made known to God; and the peace of God, which surpasses all understanding, will guard your hearts and minds through Christ Jesus." —Philippians 4:6-7

"Jesus spoke to them saying, 'Be of good cheer. It is I; do not be afraid.'" —Matthew 14:27

When Jesus spoke these words to His disciples, they were in a boat in the middle of the sea being tossed by the waves. He came walking to them on the water, and they thought it was a ghost and cried out in fear. In like fashion, when we go through the storms of life and cry out to Jesus, He is always there.

III. HELP TO OVERCOME WORRY, which can lead to anxiety and depression.

We can all worry at times. That's just human nature. But what good does worry do? Does it accomplish anything, and should we worry? The answer is quite clear: NO. Jesus makes that clear in Matthew 6:25-34. He says, "Do not worry" three times and lists several reasons why we shouldn't worry.

"Therefore I say to you, do not worry about your life, what you will eat or what you will drink; nor about your body, what you will put on. Is not life more than food and the body more than clothing? Look at the birds of the air, for they neither sow nor reap nor gather into barns; yet your heavenly Father feeds them. Are you not of more value than they? Which of you by worrying can add one cubit (eighteen inches) to his stature?

"So why do you worry about clothing? Consider the lilies of the field, how they grow: they neither toil nor spin; and yet I say to you that even Solomon in all his glory was not arrayed like one of these. Now if God so clothes the grass of the field, which today is and tomorrow is thrown into the oven, will He not much more clothe you, oh, you of little faith?

"Therefore do not worry, saying 'what shall we eat?' or 'what shall we drink?' or 'what shall we wear?' For after all these things the Gentiles seek. For your heavenly Father knows that you need all these things. But seek first the kingdom of God and His righteousness, and all these things will be added to you. Therefore do not worry about tomorrow, for tomorrow will worry about its own things. Sufficient for the day is its own trouble."

Jesus tells us how to avoid worrying: "Seek first the kingdom of God and His righteousness," and "Do not worry about tomorrow, for tomorrow will worry about its own things."

IV. HELP TO FORGIVE AND KNOW WHY WE SHOULD. Forgiveness helps the forgiver much more than the forgiven, as it brings peace and calmness, which can head off depression.

Jesus is giving His disciples a model prayer: "And forgive us our sins, as we have forgiven those who sin against us." — Matthew 6:12, NLT

Jesus continues, "If you forgive those who sin against you, your heavenly Father will forgive you. But if you refuse to forgive others, your Father will not forgive your sins." — Matthew 6:14-15, NLT

It should be noted that this does not mean believers have to ask for justification (being declared righteous in the sight of God) daily. They are justified forever from the moment of truly believing on and accepting Christ as Lord and Savior (see the last chapter of this book). But even after salvation we will make mistakes. This is more a prayer of restoring personal fellowship with God that has been hindered by sin; those who receive that forgiveness are so thankful that they also forgive others who have wronged them.[6] And, as you can tell, Jesus says forgiveness is not an option.

Here are more verses on forgiveness:

"Peter came up to Him (Jesus) and said, 'Lord, how often shall my brother sin against me, and I forgive him? Up to seven times?' Jesus said to him, 'I do not say to you, up to seven times, but up to seventy times seven.'" —Matthew 18:21-22

The apostle Paul is speaking: "And be kind to one another, tenderhearted, forgiving one another, even as God in Christ forgave you." —Ephesians 4:32

The apostle Paul also says, "Bearing with one another, and forgiving one another, if anyone has a complaint against another; even as Christ forgave you so you also must do." —Colossians 3:13

V. HELP TO KNOW WHY WE GO THROUGH TRIALS AND TRIBULATIONS: Handling trials and tribulations God's way will give us a peace that passes understanding, heading off depression.

None of us enjoys going through trials, troubles, suffering and persecutions. But it is a fact of life that these things will come. No matter who we are, whether rich or poor, educated or uneducated, live in the city or in the country, walk, ride a bike, drive a Cadillac or a Pinto and so on, trials and suffering will come. Jesus tells us, "These things I have spoken to you, that in me you may have peace. In the world you will have tribulation; but be of good cheer, I have overcome the world" (John 16:33). Jesus guarantees we will have trials and tribulation, but He clearly tells us He is our relief and our peace.

Many scriptures speak to why God allows tribulations, suffering and persecutions.

"My son, do not despise the chastening (discipline) of the Lord, nor detest His correction; for whom the Lord loves He corrects, just as a father in whom he delights." — Proverbs 3:11-12

"Now no chastening seems to be joyful for the present, but painful; nevertheless, afterward it yields the peaceable fruit of righteousness to those who have been trained by it." —Hebrews 12:11

Discipline and correction are definitely painful; but as we endure them with God's help, we are always the better for it on the other side. And, as we turn to Him, we will come closer to Him through each and every trial.

When problems and trials come we always have two options: 1. Turn away from God, and if we do this our life will begin, or continue, to crumble. 2. Turn to God which is always the right choice, and our circumstances may not immediately improve, but we will definitely be able to handle them better and move forward through them. Without a doubt, the closer we come to God through Christ, by reading and studying His Word, through prayer and through worship, public and private, the better we are able to weather the storms of life.

So then how does God say we should live during times of suffering?

"Rejoicing in hope, patient in tribulation, continuing steadfastly in prayer." —Romans 12:12

What are the benefits of trusting God and enduring through suffering?

"Blessed be the God and Father of our Lord Jesus Christ, the father of mercies and God of all comfort, who comforts us in all our tribulation, that we may be able to comfort those who are in trouble, with the comfort with which we ourselves are comforted by God" (2 Corinthians 1:3-4). We learn to comfort others.

"And not only that, but we also glory in tribulation, knowing that tribulation produces perseverance; and perseverance, character, and character, hope" (Romans 5:3-4). We have improved character and more hope.

"But may the God of all grace, who called us to His eternal glory by Christ Jesus, after you have suffered a while, perfect, establish, strengthen and settle you" (1 Peter 5:10-11). We can gain character, but there is no way around trials and tribulations to get there.

Help From God's Word

We find great encouragement for ourselves in God's Word. "Who then will condemn us? No one—for Christ Jesus died for us and was raised to life for us, and he is sitting in the place of honor at God's right hand, pleading for us. Can anything ever separate us from Christ's love? Does it mean he no longer loves us if we have trouble or calamity, or are persecuted, or hungry, or destitute, or in danger, or threatened with death?" —Romans 8:34-35, NLT

The apostle Paul continues: "No, despite all these things, overwhelming victory is ours through Christ, who loved us. And I am convinced that nothing can ever separate us from God's love. Neither death nor life, neither angels nor demons, neither our fears for today nor our worries about tomorrow—not even the powers of hell can separate us from God's love. No power in the sky above or in the earth below—indeed, nothing in all creation will ever be able to separate us from the love of God that is revealed in Christ Jesus our Lord." —Romans 8:37-39, NLT

Chapter Six
My Three Depressions And What God Taught Me

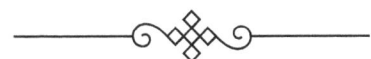

The Lord in His wisdom and because of His plan for my life has allowed me to go through three separate depressions, or depressed states. None of them was pleasant, and each one had a different trigger. In fact, each was absolutely awful, especially the first two, and all three made living each day a chore. I am not going into great detail about them as there is no reason to do that, but I will give you the gist of each one. I can't remember all the details anyway, especially of the first two. But I do definitely remember all the things God taught me and showed me, and I pray these things will help others as well.

In 1988, because of a less-than-wise financial decision or two, I caused our family to be in debt more than we should have been. Not severely so, I was thankful, but just enough to where I was worried about it. This led to anxiety and ultimately depression. Before this I had never been in a depressed state or anything close to it. I was not moody or given to worry and pretty much happy all the time. I was not pessimistic and always tried to see the good side of things.

But then something changed. It didn't seem to come on gradually, but more like one day I was fine and feeling good, and the next day a black cloud caught up with me and covered me, engulfing me in a pervasive way of thinking. All of a sudden, or so it seemed, I was not in total control of my thoughts.

Important note: as soon as I realized this, I called my doctor and told him exactly what was happening. He saw me that day and determined I needed appropriate medications; this is an important thing to do. *Get some help as quickly as possible.* (Remember the "must" paragraph and the statement from the Mayo Clinic.) As far as the medications, even though some don't work right away, as I explained, if they are necessary, the quicker you get on them the better. Some will start helping right away.

Weird and scary thoughts would speed into my mind, causing great fear and anxiety. This fueled the depressed state and seemed to make the cloud grow larger and darker. It is a vicious circle; it has a beginning, but you may not be sure why, and it will have an end. NOTE: some patients, depending on the etiology (cause) of the depression, may have to remain on medication to sustain normal thought processes. However, many like myself, may (under the direction of their doctor) be able to be weaned off their medication and do well with other practical means.

Sometimes one thought seemed to come right after another. "Where did that come from?" I would think. "Why is this in my brain? I don't believe that; I don't feel that way." Other strange thoughts would come like, "Hitler is my hero." Or I would hear of a tragedy where many people lost their lives, and the thought would come, "Should have been more." Then I would think, "But I don't feel that way. Where did that come from?" Even though I knew I didn't feel that way, the thoughts "seemed" to originate in my brain, and it scared me greatly. This obviously caused much fear, anxiety and resultant depression.

In the deepest part of the depression, before the meds started helping very much, I experienced a very specific hallucination. I would look at someone, and his head would pop off his shoulders and suspend in mid-air above him. I was not detached from reality and could clearly see that didn't happen, but at first glance that's what I saw.

As scary as that was, it wasn't the worst thing. The worst thing was the thoughts that would come for me to harm someone, either one of our sons or my beautiful wife. The thought to harm or kill myself never really came; it was always directed at them, and especially at my wife. And it scared me to death as I knew I didn't want to do that. But the thought seemed to come from me. The fear level would climb as would the anxiety, and depression thought it was winning.

But I would cry out to God, and even though I wasn't always sure He heard me, He was always there. I could see this clearer later on than I could at that moment.

I would sometimes pray, "Lord, where are You?" But relief always came as the thoughts would subside, and a subtle peace would settle in. At this point, I wanted Him to deliver me immediately from this state of mind, but that's not what happened. But He was always there, and later I could see He was in total control the whole time as I was trusting in Him and calling out to Him for help.

The scariest part of this is that since the thoughts seem to originate with you, you think maybe you want to do what they're telling you to do. You know you don't, but you wonder why they keep coming. And you can argue this point in your brain.

The truth of the matter: God showed me in the third depression that these thoughts do *not* originate with me. When our brains are not functioning properly, and our reasoning is hampered, Satan can take great advantage, and those thoughts come from him, right out of the pit. He is a spiritual being and has a certain access to our minds. He cannot make us sin; but he can lie to us, deceive us and tempt us. And that's what is going on at this point: He is the one planting those thoughts in our brains. First Peter 5:8b tells us what's going on: "Because your adversary the devil walks about like a roaring lion, seeking whom he may devour."

Satan is the real adversary. He comes to steal, kill and destroy and to train-wreck our lives. His doom is sure at the end of the age, but he's trying to take as many with him as he can to a godless eternity. In Revelation 20:10 we read, "The devil, who deceived them, was cast into the lake of fire and brimstone where the beast and the false prophet are. And they will be tormented day and night forever and ever."

Truth: What is really going on at this time is *not* that you want to harm yourself or someone else, but that you *fear* you will lose control and harm yourself or someone else. Never is it that you really want to. Don't listen to the enemy. God tells us what to do in James 4:7-8a: "Therefore submit to God. Resist the devil and he will flee from you. Draw near to God and He will draw near to you."

Depression 2 occurred in the summer of 2001, some twelve years after I was totally past the first one. With the first one I was on the prescribed medication for about seven months before tapering off under the direction of my doctor. So in 2001 I hadn't taken any meds for anxiety and depression for more than eleven years. It should be noted here that some individuals need to stay on meds for anxiety and depression all the time, depending on their actual condition and according to their doctor's directions.

I never in my wildest dream thought I would have to go through another depression, but God had more to teach me. Early that summer I was diagnosed with type II diabetes. I can't say I was overly surprised or blindsided by this as I had somewhat suspected it for probably a year. But it still hit me pretty hard. It felt like a blow between the eyes and below the belt. I was shook as I thought my eating days were over. I had heard diabetics say their doctors had told them, "If it tastes good, spit it out!"

And I didn't just love to eat—I dearly loved to eat! I had always said that being hungry was not a necessary prerequisite to eating, and being full was no real reason to quit. I was thankful I was very active, exercised and worked out a lot and was only about twenty-five to thirty pounds overweight. But that was enough extra weight, along with other factors, to help create an environment for type II diabetes.

This was also when I was diagnosed with obsessive-compulsive disorder. As I mentioned in the chapter on causes for depression, this disorder is characterized by unreasonable thoughts and fears (obsessions) that lead to repetitive behaviors (compulsions). Obviously a sidekick to depression.

I praised the Lord that this depression was not as deep as the first one. But when the weird, dominating thoughts started coming, once again I immediately saw my doctor, and he felt I needed anti-anxiety and antidepressant medication. I cannot overstate the importance of staying in close contact with your doctor, taking your meds exactly as prescribed, not stopping them without talking to your doctor and then only doing it the way he says (remember the "must" paragraph). You must be tapered off most of these meds, in order to avoid possible, severe side effects. NOTE: as previously mentioned, all meds, from aspirin to chemotherapy, can have side effects, but the percentages are usually very low. Your doctor can determine if the benefit outweighs the risk, and you can discuss that with him/her.

I had no visions of heads popping off this time nor any thoughts that Hitler was my hero; but some of the obtrusive thoughts were back. And the awful thoughts that I might harm someone or even wanted to also returned. They were not as threatening as the first time, but still scary.

Even though I was better able to handle this one, it was still tough and a very unpleasant experience. I was on medication again for about seven months before tapering off according to my doctor's orders. Each time my doctor did not consider tapering me off until I had been symptom free for several months.

Depression 3 surprised me in the spring of 2012 and, praise the Lord, was even less severe than the second one, albeit still very unpleasant. My wife and I were dealing with several family situations, with one especially much harder on her than on me because of how certain events had played out. I was doing okay. I had some anxiety but no sign of depression until one day driving home from work (a long drive) I became extremely concerned about her.

I had tried several times to call her and make sure she was ok, but she never answered. Thus my fear and anxiety levels increased. I was not fearful she would harm herself or anything like that. But what if she was laid out on the floor with a stress-related stroke or heart attack? When I arrived home, I was so thankful she was okay and on the phone with a good friend who was helping her and praying with her. But for me it was too late. The black cloud had caught up with me as I walked down the hallway toward the kitchen before finding out she was okay. Oppressive and intrusive thoughts introduced themselves to me once again. I could not believe I was in that cycle for the third time.

It was not nearly as deep or scary as either of the first two, but the fear of harming her was back. I was still not clear if it was a fear of losing control and harming her, but I definitely did *not* want to. Still scary. Inside me I knew I would never do that and that I didn't want to; but the thoughts still jumped from the dark and spooked me, sending shivers down my spine.

Immediately again I contacted my doctor who saw me quickly and prescribed the medication I needed; but this time he prescribed only an antidepressant with no anti-anxiety med included. Most antidepressants will help handle the anxiety; they're just slower in bringing it down.

Although less severe and shorter in tenure, the Lord taught me more this time than in the other two combined. I stayed on that medication for about three years at a lower dose since it helped me sleep. I tapered off it in the summer of 2015 after discussing it with my doctor. I felt I didn't need it to sleep; plus it had an annoying side effect.

** WHAT I LEARNED AND WHAT GOD TAUGHT ME **

In chapter 5 I include scriptures that let us know not only that we will go through trials and tribulations, but also why God allows them to happen. The following is a list of the lessons God taught me from my three rounds, or battles, with depression.

> The truth of His Word. Before the first depression I was not convinced of this fact. I had read the Bible my whole life, but not consistently and not necessarily looking for the truth. My Bible reading was sporadic, hit and miss, and I had no daily quiet time of prayer and reading the Word of God. Although I believed the Bible was mostly true, I was vain in my thoughts and believed I was smart enough to determine truth from non-truth in the Bible. Also at that time I wrongly believed the creation account and the theory of evolution were one and the same story, just told in different ways.

During that depression a very good friend of ours gave me a small, gold, pocket New Testament from the Gideons. As I had immediately turned to God upon realizing I was depressed, I gladly accepted it and began searching the Scriptures. I was amazed at what I found. Reading the Bible casually and inconsistently versus diligently searching the Scriptures on a daily basis with anticipation of what I could learn are two very different things.

In Deuteronomy 4:29 we read, "But from there you will seek the Lord your God, and you will find Him if you seek Him with all your heart and with all your soul." And Proverbs 8:17 reminds us, "I love those who love me, and those who seek me diligently will find me." Through seeking God in His Word and in prayer and through a Bible study at our church, God showed me without any shadow of doubt that His Word, the Holy Bible, is the inspired, inerrant, authoritative Word of God as I describe in chapter 4.

> Also during that time God impressed upon me that I should be more faithful to serve Him. My wife and I had been active in serving in our church, teaching Sunday school and singing in the choir, and I had also served as an elder. But this was different; it was somehow deeper. I first thought He wanted me to become a pastor. As I continued to seek Him, though, it became clear that wasn't it.

One day He made it very clear to me, and all doubt about what He was calling me to do vanished. It was as if He stood before me and said, "You are to be a Gideon!"

I replied, "Lord, who are You talking to? I'm the only one here!"

"To you," He answered, and that ended the discussion.

Our best friends were in the Gideon ministry. As I said earlier, this is a ministry with only one purpose, and that is to see that every person on earth has an opportunity to accept Jesus Christ as Lord and Savior. We accomplish that by the distribution and placement of God's Word and by personal evangelism.

I saw no burning bush in the room that day, nor did I hear an audible voice. But I might as well have because what He spoke to my spirit went straight to my heart and penetrated my innermost being. I went from wondering what He wanted me to do to knowing without a shadow of a doubt the path He had chosen for me.

When I told my wife, she felt the call as well, and we signed up that very week. The Lord has truly blessed us in this ministry since we joined in November 1988, and He continues to do so each and every day. Praise the Lord!

> Also during that first depression God began to show me how big He is and how small Satan is in contrast. Satan is a powerful foe, and we must be on our guard and trust the Lord for protection. But in comparison to God he is small, very small. In the Bible in the book of Job we can clearly see that Satan can only do what God allows him to do. God first tells Satan he can touch everything of Job's except his body or his health. Job remains faithful to God after that, so Satan complains to God that Job wouldn't remain faithful if he lost his health. So God allows Satan to touch his health, but not take his life. Job still remains faithful to God, although he becomes a pretty good complainer. In the end, God restores everything Job had and even more.

Through the deepest part of that depression I sometimes felt as if God was not around, that my prayers were falling on dull ears. Nothing was further from the truth. Although I couldn't see it clearly then, later I began to see how God had answered my prayer every time. He was always there; He was always in control. God is sovereign, and the devil has no power over Him. But to build our faith in Him and for all the other reasons listed in chapter 5, God allows us to go through suffering and hard times. Like Job, we must endure and trust the Lord even when He is silent.

> God also showed me where the real battle is being fought, who the real enemy is and how we should dress for the battle.

> A final word: Be strong in the Lord and in his mighty power. Put on all of God's armor so that you will be able to stand firm against all strategies of the devil. For we are not fighting against flesh-and-blood enemies, but against evil rulers and authorities of the unseen world, against mighty powers in this dark world, and against evil spirits in the heavenly places.
>
> Therefore, put on every piece of God's armor so you will be able to resist the enemy in the time of evil. Then after the battle you will still be standing firm. Stand your ground, putting on the belt of truth and the body armor of God's righteousness. For shoes, put on the peace that comes from the Good News so that you will be fully prepared. In addition to all of these, hold

up the shield of faith to stop the fiery arrows of the devil. Put on salvation as your helmet, and take the sword of the Spirit, which is the word of God.

Pray in the Spirit at all times and on every occasion. Stay alert and be persistent in your prayers for all believers everywhere (Ephesians 6:10-18, NLT).

(See Chapter 7 on how to be right with God in God's eyes.)

The following is a song the Lord gave me describing this process, from the above verses and from James 4:7.

THE SWORD OF THE SPIRIT

The enemy came, in the middle of the night;
He was armed and ready, lookin' for a fight.
His weapons were drawn; there was fire in his eyes.
His breath was hot as he breathed forth lies.

I was not prepared for his attack.
My sword was dusty; my shield was cracked.
They'd lain on a shelf for way too long;
Hadn't been used, couldn't make me strong.

He hit me low; he hit me high.
I wanted to run; I wanted to cry.
Wounded and weak, I was covered in gloom.
I thought he laughed as he left the room.

CHORUS:
Go to My Word, I heard the Lord say.
It will light your path and increase your faith.
It is the truth to tell right from wrong.
The Word of God is the sword of the Spirit that will make you strong.

We wrestle not against flesh and blood
But with spiritual wickedness from up above.
So put on the whole armor of God,
And your feet with the gospel of peace will be shod.

Stand with the truth up around your waist
And on your chest the righteous breastplate.
To quench those fiery darts you must take
And place before you the shield of faith.

Having on the helmet of salvation,
Praying always with prayer and supplication;
And when the enemy comes you will see
You can resist him, and he will flee.

CHORUS:

Go to My Word, I heard the Lord say.

It will light your path and increase your faith.

It is the truth to tell right from wrong.

The Word of God is the sword of the Spirit that will make you strong.

> As I stated before, Satan cannot make us sin; he does not have the freedom or power to do that. But he can tempt us, lie to us and deceive us. In 2 Timothy 2:25-26 we are told to "gently instruct those who oppose the truth. Perhaps God will change those people's hearts, and they will learn the truth. Then they will come to their senses and escape the devil's trap. For they have been held captive by him to do whatever he wants" (NLT).

Those intrusive thoughts we mistakenly think come from us—to harm or kill us or someone else or to do other such hideous acts—as I said, *do not come from us.* They come right out of the pit from the devil himself. Remember: he is a spiritual being and has a certain access to our thoughts. Don't listen to him. He is a liar and a deceiver. I quoted Revelation 20:10 earlier; it starts out, "The devil, who deceives them. . . ." And then in John 8:44 Jesus is talking: "You are of your father the devil, and the desires of your father you want to do. He was a murderer from the beginning, and does not stand in the truth, because there is no truth in him. When he speaks a lie, he speaks from his own resources, for he is a liar and the father of it."

> He showed me I need to send all fears and worries up to Him. Remember the psalmist's words: "I sought the Lord, and He heard me, and delivered me from all my fears" (Psalm 34:4), and "Cast your burden on the Lord, and He shall sustain you" (Psalm 55:22a). Think about these promises too: "Casting all your care upon Him, for He cares for you" (1 Peter 5:7), and "Come to Me, all you who labor and are heavy laden, and I will give you rest" (Matthew 11:28).

It is very clear from God's Word that He wants us to send all cares, burdens, fears, anxieties and worries up to Him. He is much more able to handle them than we are. When we send them up to Him, we must believe and trust that He will help us. It doesn't mean that what's causing the fear will immediately disappear; but our ability to handle it will get better, and this will help us. And if it comes back, the fear and anxiety may start; but if we remember we've given it to Him it will disappear.

> I truly learned He is always there. This happened during the third depression; one night I awakened, and fear was present. I was afraid I would lose control and do something awful to my dear wife, who was sleeping comfortably next to me. Right then I wasn't clear that these were not my thoughts. The anxiety level was quickly running up the scale and was about to ring the buzzer on the top when it got worse. My arms and hands began to tingle, and by what seemed a

supernatural force my hands were moving slowly toward her neck—but I wasn't doing it.

I gasped in my heart and mind. How could this be? I told myself, "I don't want to do that! How could I do it? I won't do that!" But it seemed as if I didn't have full control. With fear gripping every ounce of me, I cried out to God, "O Lord, help me. I need help! Please help me!"

Instantly He was there, and the Holy Spirit spoke to my mind: "The anxiety is causing your arms and hands to tingle. It is just the anxiety."

"Just the anxiety," I repeated to myself and started to relax all over. I knew God was with me and protecting me and her. The tingling went away as I continued thanking and praising Him for His protection and for always being there. That was the only time it happened to that degree, when I thought my hands were moving and did move slightly. Pretty soon I drifted back to sleep. I had learned a huge lesson. God is always there.

> Those are not my thoughts. As I have previously stated, those intrusive, ugly thoughts don't come from us; they come right out of the pit from the devil. I heard a statement one time that said, "If Satan reminds you of your past, remind him of his future!" Remember: Revelation 20:10 tells us Satan will be cast into the lake of fire and brimstone and be tormented day and night forever and ever. So now when those intrusive, oppressive thoughts come, I just declare, "Not my thoughts!" And I picture Satan going into the lake of fire, and he cannot

do anything about it. He is stuck there forever. Amen. Then I quote the Scriptures (see next bullet point).

Since I'm not in a depressed state of mind now, praise the Lord, those oppressive thoughts don't come. But still a stray thought I know is not mine can swing through, and I will declare, "Not my thought!" I also do that when temptations come (see next bullet point).

> How to battle bad thoughts and temptations. We should oppose bad thoughts and temptations the same way Jesus did when Satan was tempting Him to sin, as we read in Matthew 4:1-11. With each temptation the devil hurls at Jesus, Jesus quotes Scripture to counter it. With the first temptation Jesus quotes Deuteronomy 8:3c; with the second, Psalm 91:11-12; and with the third, Deuteronomy 6:16a. Jesus, being all God and all man, could have easily told the devil to buzz off and that he had no power over Him. But He didn't do that; instead He gave us an example of how to defeat the devil.

But obviously we must know the Scriptures to do that. Psalm 119:11 tells us, "Your Word I have hidden in my heart, that I might not sin against you." God tells us in His Word to hide His Word in our heart, to memorize the Scriptures, so as not to be taken captive by the devil to do his will.

Toward the end of the last depression, when the devil would try to deceive me into harming my wife, I learned to quote Psalm 101:4b. I would say, "It is written, 'I will know nothing of evil.'" Then I would declare, "In Jesus' name!" And the thought would disappear, praise the Lord.

I'm thankful I don't have much of that anymore; but temptations do come, and quoting Scripture is a good way not to give in to them.

Unfortunately, foul language is rampant in our society, and two good verses to quote if those kinds of thoughts arrive in our brains are: "Let no corrupt word proceed out of your mouth" (Ephesians 4:29a), and "But now you yourselves are to put off all these: anger, wrath, malice, blasphemy, filthy language out of your mouth" (Colossians 3:8). Precede it with "It is written," and end it with "In Jesus' name."

> No evaluation necessary. Don't evaluate or be judgmental when thoughts come to your mind about every little thing someone says or does. The Lord showed me I was over-evaluating many things and that it wasn't right. Obviously, sometimes it's proper to speak up and offer advice, but we can all be overly judgmental at times. I believe over-evaluation is a characteristic of the OCD brain; we can think our way is the best and only way. Judgmental thoughts can be very destructive if verbalized into criticism toward another person.

The Word of God is very clear in a number of Scripture verses that we are not to be judgmental. For example, in Romans 14:10 the apostle Paul says, "But why do you judge your brother? Or why do you show contempt for your brother? For we will all stand before the judgment seat of Christ." And in verses 12-13a of the same chapter he says, "So then each of us shall give an account of himself to God. Therefore let us not judge one another anymore." Jesus put it like this in Matthew 7:1-2: "Judge not, that you be not judged. For with what judgment you judge, you will be judged; and with the measure you use, it will be measured back to you."

> The interpretation of the dream. In chapter 1 I shared a recurring dream I had as a child. All through the years I had no idea if the dream had an interpretation or not. Only after the third depression did God reveal to me the interpretation of the dream.

The lumberjack chopping off the logs is Satan, who is consistently hurling trials and tribulations my way. As the logs varied in size, the size of the log had to do with the size of the trial, and I am thankful to the Lord for more little ones than big ones. Since none of the logs actually made a direct hit on me, this indicated none of the trials was as severe as they could have been because in every one I turned to the Lord for help. Obviously, turning away from the Lord would have brought a direct hit and much more severe consequences. As the logs never stopped coming, I know the trials will never stop either. As my paddling against the air did very little to move me out of the path of the logs, so my own feeble efforts alone would not have moved me through the trial successfully. Only God's supernatural intervention kept me from any direct hits by the logs and by the trials. Praise the Lord. Praise His name, the name of Jesus!

Chapter Seven
God Loves You

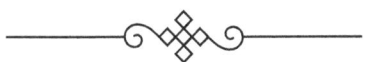

** **Of eternal importance: How to be right with God** **

What is God's will for you? That you spend eternity with Him! "The Lord is not slack concerning His promise, as some count slackness, but is longsuffering toward us, not willing that any should perish but that all should come to repentance" (2 Peter 3:9).

> God loves you. "For God so loved the world that He gave His only begotten Son, that whoever believes in Him should not perish but have everlasting life" (John 3:16).

> What separates us from God? Our sin. "The next day John saw Jesus coming toward him, and said, 'Behold, the Lamb of God who takes away the sin of the world!'" (John 1:29). Also, "For the wages of sin is death, but the gift of God is eternal life in Christ Jesus our Lord" (Romans 6:23).

> Who has sinned? Everyone. "As it is written: There is none righteous, no, not one" (Romans 3:10). Also, "For all have sinned and fall short of the glory of God" (Romans 3:23).

> Why did Jesus say He came? "For the Son of Man has come to seek and to save that which was lost" (Luke 19:10).

> What are we saved from? Jesus said, "So it will be at the end of the age. The angels will come forth, separate the wicked from among the just, and cast them into the furnace of fire. There will be wailing and gnashing of teeth" (Matthew 13:49-50). Also, "Anyone not found written in the Book of Life was cast into the lake of fire" (Revelation 20:15). Jesus tells of the unsaved going to a place "where their worm does not die, and the fire is not quenched" (Mark 9:42-48). Not a place you want to spend eternity!

> God's remedy for sin. "For God so loved the world that He gave His only begotten Son, that whoever believes in Him should not perish but have everlasting life" (John 3:16). Also, "For the wages of sin is death, but the gift of God is eternal life in Christ Jesus our Lord" (Romans 6:23). Further, "But God demonstrates His own love toward us, in that while we were still sinners, Christ died for us" (Romans 5:8).

> How are we saved? "If you confess with your mouth the Lord Jesus and believe in your heart that God has raised Him from the dead, you will be saved. For with the heart one believes unto righteousness, and with the mouth confession is made unto salvation" (Romans 10:9-10). And "by grace you have been saved through faith, and that not of yourselves; it

is the gift of God, not of works, lest anyone should boast" (Ephesians 2:8-9). Grace is unmerited favor.

> Who can be saved? "When His disciples heard it, they were greatly astonished, saying, 'Who then can be saved?' But Jesus looked at them and said to them, 'With men this is impossible, but with God all things are possible'" (Matthew 19:25-26). Jesus said, "Behold, I stand at the door and knock. If anyone hears My voice and opens the door, I will come in to him and dine with him, and he with Me" (Revelation 3:20). The apostle Paul wrote, "For whoever calls on the name of the Lord shall be saved" (Romans 10:13).

> Is there another way? No. "Jesus said to him, 'I am the way, the truth, and the life. No one comes to the Father except through me'" (John 14:6). To say there is another way is to call Jesus a liar!

> My decision to receive Christ as my Savior. If you can pray something like the prayer you see below and truly mean it in your heart, being sorry for your sins, and trust Christ alone as your Lord and Savior, you can know for certain you will go to heaven when you die. This is not a magic prayer; you must mean it sincerely in your heart.

> Lord God, I confess to You that I am a sinner. I am sorry for my sins, and I believe the Lord Jesus Christ's death on the cross and resurrection from the dead cleared my sins. I accept Him and confess Him as my Lord and my Savior. Amen!

NAME_____

DATE_____

> Assurance as a believer. "If you confess with your mouth the Lord Jesus and believe in your heart that God raised Him from the dead, you will be saved" (Romans 10:9). Jesus said, "Most assuredly, I say to you, he who hears My word and believes in Him who sent Me has everlasting life, and shall not come into judgment, but has passed from death into life" (John 5:24). He also said, "But these are written that you may believe that Jesus is the Christ, the Son of God, and believing you may have life in His name" (John 20:31).

> After you receive Christ as Savior, I recommend you find a Bible-teaching and -preaching church—one that teaches and preaches the absolute truth of God's Word. There you can be discipled, and grow in your newfound faith in Christ. "But grow in the grace and knowledge of our Lord and Savior Jesus Christ" (2 Peter 3:18). To Him be the glory both now and forever. Amen.

References

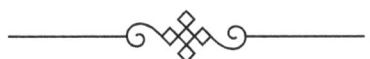

All scriptures quoted are from the Holy Bible, New King James Version, Copyright © 1982 Thomas Nelson. All rights reserved. Scriptures marked NLT are taken from The Holy Bible, New Living Translation, copyright 1996, 2004, 2007 by Tyndale House Foundation. Tyndale House Publishers Inc. Carol Stream, IL 60188. All rights reserved.

1 "Understanding Depression and Bipolar Disorder," Institute for Natural Resources (INR), INR Seminar, First Edition (8-14), P.O. Box 5757, Concord, CA 94524, 2014.

2 *The Jeremiah Study Bible*, David Jeremiah Inc., Worthy Publishing, Worthy Media Inc., 2013.

3 "The Wonderful Word of God, History Written in Advance", Bible Hour Message, Bryan Hughes, senior pastor, Grace Bible Church, 3625 South 19th Street, Bozeman, MT 59718, Oct. 2015.

4 Marc Estes, Making Life Count, marcestes.com, Article "The Bible is Indestructible" March 12, 2010.

5 Mayo Clinic, mayoclinic.org

6 *The ESV Study Bible*, English Standard Version (ESV), Copyright © 2008 by Crossway Bibles, a publishing ministry of Good News Publishers. All rights reserved.

7 *The Merriam-Webster Dictionary*, merriam-webster.com

www.ingramcontent.com/pod-product-compliance
Ingram Content Group UK Ltd.
Pitfield, Milton Keynes, MK11 3LW, UK
UKHW041949230426
12048UKWH00008B/218